Table of Contents

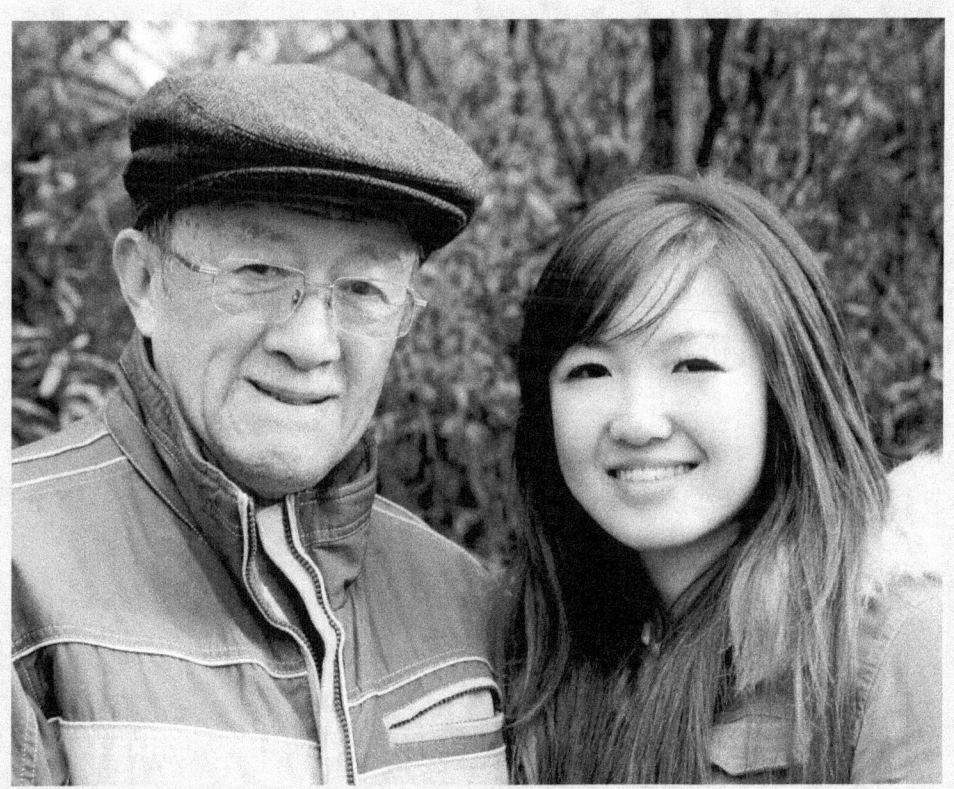

Many older adults and their families are faced with Alzheimer's disease. It's important to know the signs of the disease and where to get help.

Introduction

Many older people forget someone's name or misplace things from time to time. This kind of forgetfulness is normal. But, forgetting how to get home, getting confused in places a person knows well, or asking questions over and over can be signs of a more serious problem. The person may have **Alzheimer's disease** (pronounced **Allz**-high-merz duh-**zeez**). It is a disease of the brain that begins slowly and gets worse over time.

> ## This booklet will help you learn about Alzheimer's disease:
>
> - what it is
> - signs of the disease
> - when it is important to see your doctor
> - treatment
> - research studies
> - how to get help caring for a person with the disease

Tips about using this booklet

Use the Table of Contents to help you find things quickly. Also, we put some medical terms in bold, such as **Alzheimer's disease.** You can find how to say these words and what they mean in the "Words to know" section on page 19.

Helen's story

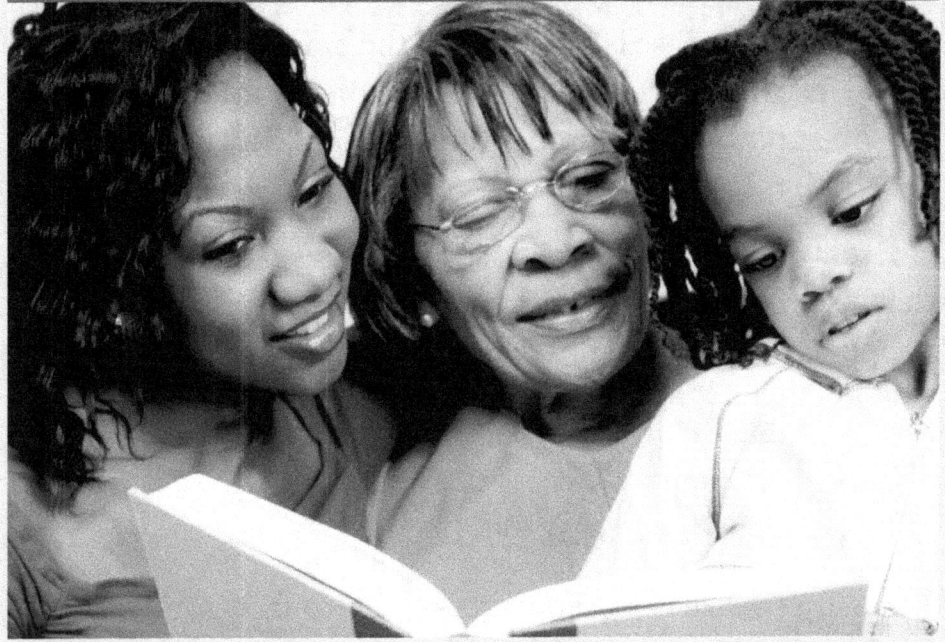

I have Alzheimer's disease. It took me a long time before I could even say the words. When the doctor first told me, I felt like my life was over. For a while, I was depressed. My doctor told me about medicine I could take. She said it would slow down my memory loss for a while. I know it's not a cure. Still, it feels good to do something.

My family has been wonderful. They're helping me plan for the care I'll need. I have decided to take each day as it comes. I want to live my life as fully as I can.

What is Alzheimer's disease?

Alzheimer's disease is an illness of the brain. It causes large numbers of nerve cells in the brain to die. This affects a person's ability to remember things, think clearly, and use good judgment.

Doctors don't know what causes the disease. They do know that most of the time it begins after age 60. Nearly half of people age 85 and older may have Alzheimer's.

What happens when a person has Alzheimer's disease?

Alzheimer's disease often starts slowly. In fact, some people don't know they have it. They blame their forgetfulness on old age. However, over time, their memory problems get more serious.

People with Alzheimer's disease have trouble doing everyday things like driving a car, cooking a meal, or paying bills. They may get lost easily and find even simple things confusing. Some people become worried, angry, or violent.

As the illness gets worse, most people with Alzheimer's disease need someone to take care of all their needs, including feeding and bathing. Some people with Alzheimer's live at home with a caregiver. Other people with the disease live in a nursing home.

What are the signs of Alzheimer's disease?

It's important to know the signs of Alzheimer's disease. If you know the signs, you can get help right away. Some signs of the disease are listed here:

Early signs

- finding it hard to remember things
- asking the same questions over and over
- having trouble paying bills or solving simple math problems
- getting lost
- losing things or putting them in odd places

Later signs

- forgetting how to brush your teeth or comb your hair
- being confused about time, people, and places
- forgetting the names of common things such as a desk, house, or apple
- wandering away from home

Mild cognitive impairment

Some older people have a condition called **mild cognitive impairment**, or MCI. It can be an early sign of Alzheimer's. But, not everyone with MCI will develop Alzheimer's disease. People with MCI can still take care of themselves and do their normal activities. MCI memory problems may include:

- losing things often

- forgetting to go to events or appointments

- having more trouble coming up with words than other people the same age.

If you have MCI, it's important to see your doctor or specialist every 6 to 12 months. Ask him or her to check for changes in your memory and thinking.

Differences between Alzheimer's disease and normal aging

Use the chart below to help you understand the differences between Alzheimer's disease and the normal signs of aging.

Alzheimer's disease	Normal aging
Making poor judgments and decisions a lot of the time	Making a bad decision once in a while
Problems taking care of monthly bills	Missing a monthly payment
Losing track of the date or time of year	Forgetting which day it is and remembering it later
Trouble having a conversation	Sometimes forgetting which word to use
Misplacing things often and being unable to find them	Losing things from time to time

Rita's story

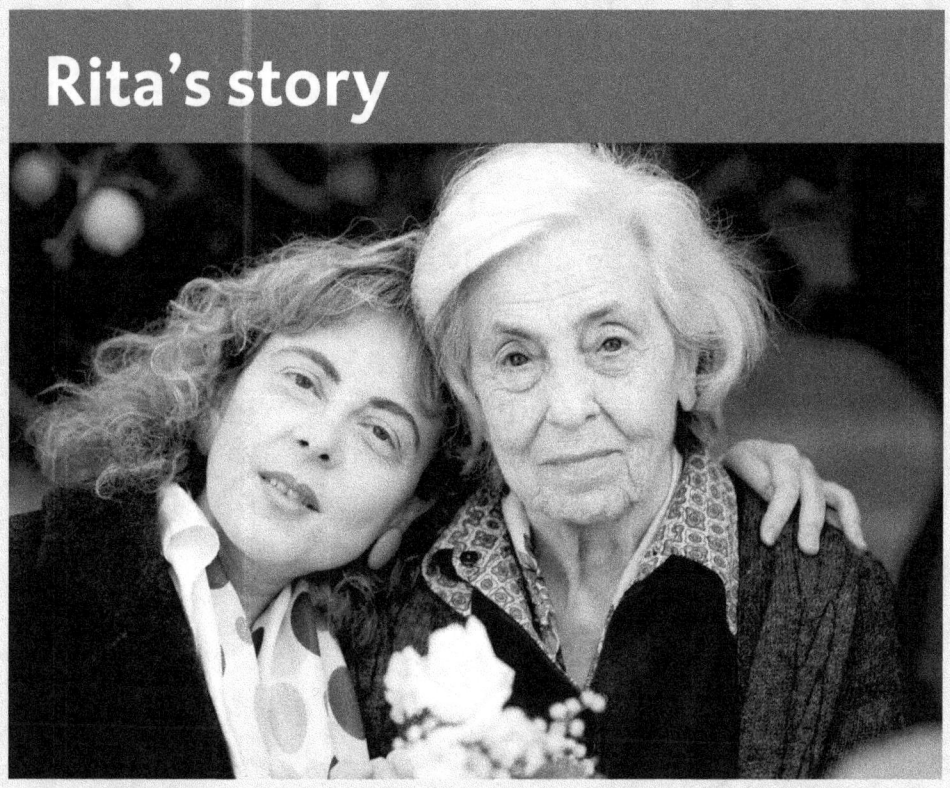

A few months ago, my mother started having trouble remembering things. Sometimes, she couldn't find the right words. Then, she got lost on her way home from the store. I knew something was wrong. I talked with my mom, and we decided to see her doctor.

The doctor asked about the changes we had seen and did a medical exam. He also changed one of Mom's medicines to see if that would make a difference. And, he suggested that she see a specialist who could test her memory and thinking skills. He said it was good that she came in now instead of waiting so we could start figuring out what the problem might be.

When should you see your doctor?

If you or someone in your family thinks your forgetfulness is getting in the way of your normal routine, it's time to see your doctor. **Seeing the doctor when you first start having memory problems can help you find out what's causing your forgetfulness.** If you have Alzheimer's, finding the disease early gives you and your family more time to plan for your treatment and care.

Your doctor or a specialist may do the following things to find out if you have Alzheimer's disease:

- give you a medical check-up

- ask questions about your family's health

- ask how well you can do everyday things like driving, shopping for food, and paying bills

- talk with someone in your family about your memory problems

- test your memory, problem-solving, counting, and language skills

- check your blood and urine, and do other medical tests

- do brain scans that show pictures of your brain

Linda's story

My neighbor Rose was always very active. She liked gardening and helping out at the local grade school. She and her husband Bob enjoyed dancing and spending time with their grandkids. After Bob passed away 2 years ago, something changed. Rose began spending a lot of time alone at home. She seemed more and more confused.

I was worried that Rose had Alzheimer's disease and convinced her to see a doctor. It turns out that she doesn't have Alzheimer's. Depression and not eating well were causing her problems. After seeing a counselor, taking medicine, and eating better, she seems less confused and more like herself.

What are other causes of memory problems?

Some medical conditions cause confusion and forgetfulness. The signs may look like Alzheimer's disease, but they are caused by other problems. Here are medical conditions that can cause serious memory problems:

- bad reaction to certain medicines

- emotional problems such as **depression**

- not eating enough healthy foods

- too few vitamins and minerals in your body

- drinking too much alcohol

- blood clots or tumors in the brain

- head injury, such as concussion from a fall or accident

- kidney, liver, or thyroid problems

These medical conditions are serious and need to be treated. Once you get treatment, your confusion and forgetfulness should go away.

Rick's story

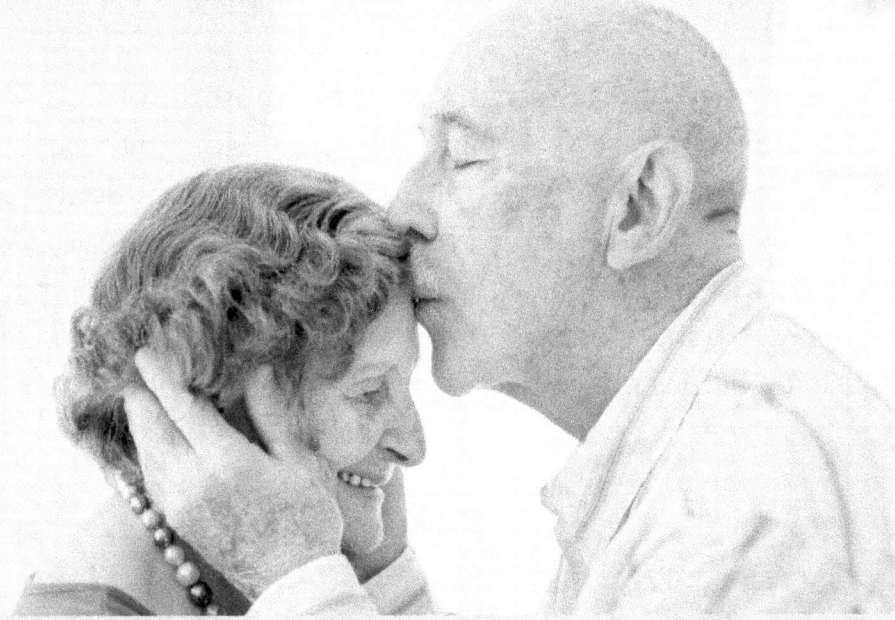

My wife Jenny was diagnosed with Alzheimer's disease a few years ago. She's been taking medicine for her memory problems. It's helped some, but now she seems to be getting worse.

We talked with the doctor. He's going to change her medicine and see if that helps. We both know there is no cure, but we do want more time together.

Are there treatments for Alzheimer's disease?

There are medicines that can treat the symptoms of Alzheimer's disease. But, there is no cure. Most of these medicines work best for people in the early or middle stages of the disease. For example, they can keep your memory loss from getting worse for a time. Other medicines may help if you have trouble sleeping, or are worried and depressed. All these medicines may have side effects and may not work for everyone.

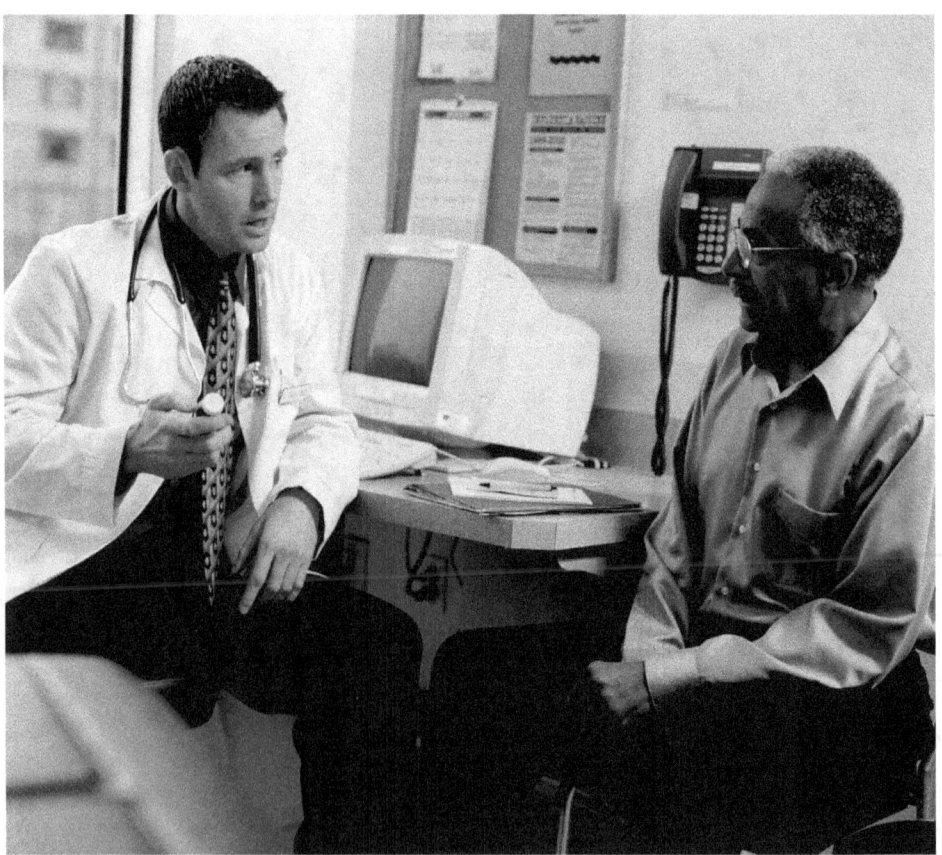

Some medicines can help treat the symptoms of Alzheimer's disease.

Ed's story

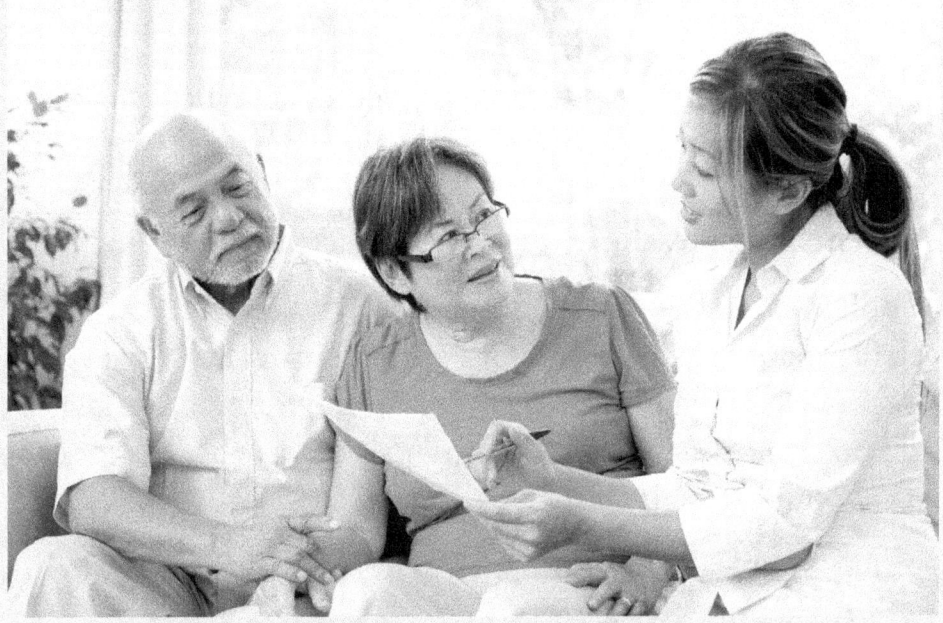

My nephew told me about an Alzheimer's disease study at a nearby research center. I don't have memory problems now, but the disease runs in my family, so I worry about it. I called to find out about the study. The nurse asked me some questions about myself and my family health history to see if I could join. Later, my wife and I set up a time to go to the research center.

Taking part in the study has been interesting. Research like this could help in finding new treatments or even someday preventing Alzheimer's. Being part of a study is important to help my family and others in the future.

What about research on Alzheimer's disease?

Researchers are doing studies with people who have different kinds of memory problems to find new and better ways to treat the disease. They also are looking at how to prevent Alzheimer's, slow the disease, and reduce its symptoms.

People with Alzheimer's disease, MCI, or a family history of Alzheimer's may be able to take part in **clinical trials**, a type of research study. Healthy people with no memory problems and no family history of Alzheimer's also may be able to take part in clinical trials.

Joining a clinical trial or other research study is a way to help fight Alzheimer's disease.

To find out more about clinical trials and studies:

- Call the Alzheimer's Disease Education and Referral Center (ADEAR) at **1-800-438-4380.** It's a free call.

- Visit the ADEAR Center website at **www.nia.nih.gov/Alzheimers.**

- Check out **www.ClinicalTrials.gov.**

John's story

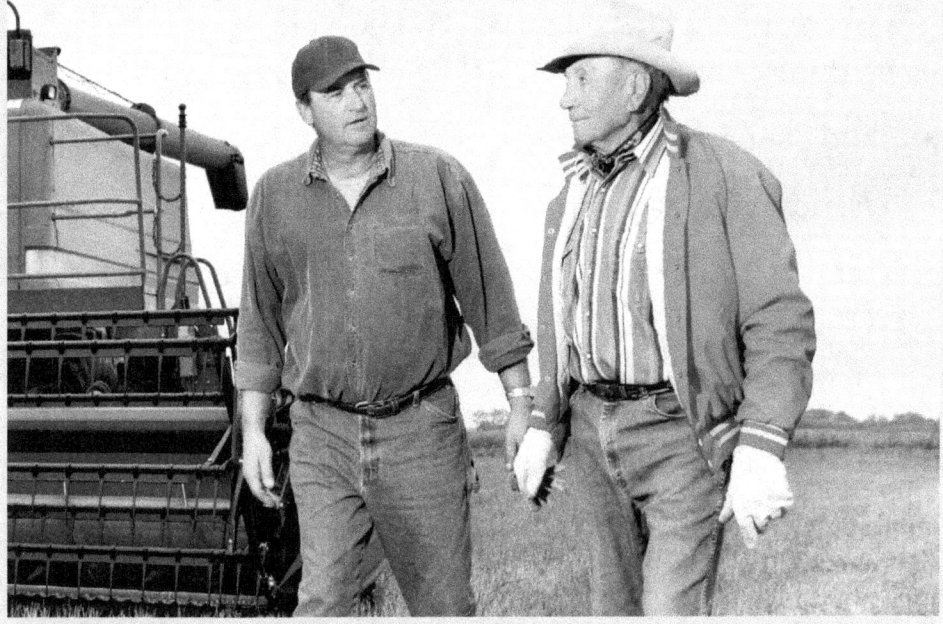

My neighbor's mom has Alzheimer's disease. I never thought it would happen to someone in my family. I was upset and worried when I found out my father had the disease. I had so many questions. What is Alzheimer's disease? Can it be treated? How is the disease going to affect my father? Will I be able to care for him? Where can I go for help? In time, I found information on the Internet and by calling Alzheimer's groups.

Is there help for caregivers?

Yes, there is help for caregivers. You don't have to do everything yourself. See the list below for ways to get help.

- Find a support group.

- Use adult day care services.

- Get help from a local home health care agency.

- Contact local and national groups for information about Alzheimer's disease.

Be sure to check out pages 17 and 18 for groups and services that can help you.

Coping as a caregiver

If you are caring for someone with Alzheimer's disease, you may have many different feelings. Sometimes, taking care of the person with Alzheimer's makes you feel good because you are providing love and comfort. At other times, it can be overwhelming. You may see changes in the person that are hard to understand and cope with.

Each day brings new challenges. You may find yourself dealing with problem behaviors or just trying to get through the day. You may not even realize how much you have taken on, because the changes can happen slowly over time.

Take care of yourself

Taking care of yourself is one of the most important things you can do as a caregiver. You could:

- ask friends and family to help out

- do things you enjoy and spend time with friends

- take short breaks

- eat healthy foods and get exercise

Taking these actions can bring you some relief. It also may help keep you from getting ill or depressed.

Summary—What you need to know

- Know the signs of Alzheimer's disease.

- See a doctor right away if you are worried about your memory problems.

- Take medicines to help treat the symptoms of Alzheimer's disease. Right now, there is no cure.

- Think about joining a clinical trial if you are healthy or if you have Alzheimer's disease.

- Get help if you are caring for someone with Alzheimer's.

See your doctor if you are worried about your memory or think you might have Alzheimer's disease. It's important to find out what is causing your memory problems.

Where can you get more information?

Contact the following groups to learn more about Alzheimer's disease. They can help you find information, support groups, and services. They also can give you information about clinical trials and other research studies.

Alzheimer's Disease Education and Referral Center (ADEAR)

P.O. Box 8250
Silver Spring, MD 20907-8250
Phone: **1-800-438-4380**
Website: **www.nia.nih.gov/Alzheimers**

This Center provides information on:

- diagnosing Alzheimer's disease

- treating Alzheimer's symptoms

- caring for the person with the disease

- meeting the needs of caregivers

- finding long-term care for the person with Alzheimer's

- taking part in Alzheimer's disease research

ADEAR Center staff can refer you to local and national resources. The Center is a service of the National Institute on Aging, part of the Federal Government's National Institutes of Health.

Alzheimer's Association
Phone: **1-800-272-3900**
Website: **www.alz.org**

The Alzheimer's Association is a nonprofit group offering information and support services to people with Alzheimer's disease and their caregivers and families. The Alzheimer's Association also sponsors research. Call or visit their website to find out where to get help in your area.

Alzheimer's Foundation of America
Phone: **1-866-232-8484**
Website: **www.alzfdn.org**

This nonprofit group serves people with Alzheimer's disease and their caregivers and families. Services include a toll-free hotline, publications, and online resources.

Eldercare Locator
Phone: **1-800-677-1116**
Website: **www.eldercare.gov**

The Eldercare Locator helps families find resources in their community, such as home care, adult day care, and nursing homes. Contact them to learn about services in your area. The Eldercare Locator is a service of the Administration on Aging. It is funded by the Federal Government.

Words to know

Alzheimer's disease
(pronounced **Allz**-high-merz duh-**zeez**)
A disease that causes large numbers of nerve cells in the brain to die. This affects a person's ability to remember things, think clearly, and use good judgment. The symptoms begin slowly and get worse over time.

Clinical trial
(pronounced **klin**-uh-kuhl **try**-uhl)
A research study to find out if new treatments are safe and effective. Healthy people and people with Alzheimer's disease can choose to take part in a clinical trial.

Depression
(pronounced dee-**presh**-uhn)
A serious medical illness that can be treated. Some signs of depression are:

- feeling sad for more than a few weeks at a time
- having trouble sleeping
- losing interest in things you like to do

Depression can cause people to be confused and forgetful.

Mild cognitive impairment
(pronounced mild **kog**-ni-tiv im-**pair**-ment)
Also called MCI. It is a medical condition that causes people to have more memory problems than other people their age. The signs of MCI are not as severe as those of Alzheimer's disease.

www.ingramcontent.com/pod-product-compliance
Lightning Source LLC
Chambersburg PA
CBHW080405290526
45790CB00009BA/3705